Journey to a Better You:

Strategies for Long-Term Weight Loss Success

by

Maximilian Blake

Introduction

Losing weight is a journey that can be challenging, but the rewards - better health, increased energy, and greater self-confidence - are well worth it. However, for many people, navigating the complexities of weight loss can be daunting, especially with so much conflicting information available online.

This book is designed to be your guide on your journey to healthier you. Whether you're just starting out and looking to lose a few pounds or seeking long-term weight loss success, you'll find valuable information, practical strategies, and motivational advice to help you reach your goals.

In this book, we'll explore the key components of successful weight loss, including nutrition, exercise, mindset, and self-care, as well as strategies for overcoming common obstacles. We'll also provide you with actionable tips, recipes, and exercises that you can implement right away to start your weight loss journey on the right foot.

At the end of the day, we believe that healthy living is not a one-size-fits-all endeavor, and the weight loss journey is just that - a journey. Our goal is to provide you with the knowledge, inspiration, and tools to help you achieve success in a way that feels sustainable and authentic to you.

So, are you ready to embark on the journey to a better you? Let's get started!

Chapter 1

Why Losing Weight Matters

Losing weight is a goal that many people have, but it's important to understand why it matters beyond simply fitting into a smaller clothing size or looking better in a swimsuit. In fact, there are several critical reasons that you should prioritize weight loss as part of your overall health and wellness plan.

Obesity has become a significant health concern for adults and children alike. According to the Centers for Disease Control and Prevention, more than one-third of adults in the United States are obese, which means they have a body mass index (BMI) of 30 or higher. Being overweight or obese is linked to a variety of health problems, including heart disease, diabetes, joint pain and mobility issues, and even certain types of cancer.

But the good news is that even modest weight loss can make a significant difference in your health outcomes. Losing just 5 to 10 percent of your body weight can reduce your risk of developing chronic diseases, improve your mobility and energy levels, and even boost your mood and mental outlook.

Developing a comprehensive weight loss plan that prioritizes not just a number on the scale, but a holistic approach to health, is critical to achieving your goals and sustaining them over the long term. This involves making healthy choices in terms of your diet, incorporating regular exercise into your routine, and addressing the underlying mental and emotional factors that can contribute to unhealthy behaviors.

In this book, we'll delve into the science of weight loss and provide a roadmap for creating your own personalized weight loss plan. But first, it's important to take a step back and reflect on why weight loss matters to you personally. What motivates you to make the changes necessary to improve your health and wellbeing? What barriers have prevented you from achieving success in the past?

As we explore each facet of successful weight loss, from nutrition and exercise to mindset and motivation, it's important to stay connected to your personal "why." Understanding the reasons behind your weight loss goals can help you stay focused on the big picture and celebrate your successes along the way.

By the end of this book, you'll have the tools and knowledge you need to create a sustainable, comprehensive approach to weight loss that works for your lifestyle, preferences, and unique

body and mindset. But for now,
let's dive into the science of
weight loss and explore how your
body and mind respond to
changes in diet and exercise.

Chapter 2

Understanding the Science of Weight Loss

Losing weight is often thought of as a matter of simple math: eat fewer calories than you burn, and the pounds will melt away. But the reality is much more complex than that. Understanding the science of weight loss can help you make informed decisions about your nutrition and exercise plan and create a sustainable approach to long-term success.

At its core, weight loss requires creating a calorie deficit. This means that you need to burn more calories than you consume in order to lose weight. However, not all calories are created equal when it comes to weight loss. For example, a calorie from a piece of candy won't affect your body in the same way as a calorie from a vegetable.

To create a sustainable calorie deficit, it's important to focus on nutrient-dense, whole foods that provide your body with the energy and nutrients it needs to function optimally. These foods typically have fewer calories per serving than processed or high-fat foods, but they can also help you feel fuller and more satisfied, so you're less likely to overeat. Along with calorie balance, there are several other factors to consider when it comes to weight loss. One of the most important is your metabolism, which is the process by which your body converts food into energy. Your metabolism can vary based on a variety of factors, including genetics, age, and hormone levels.

Several hormones are key players in the weight loss process. Leptin is a hormone that signals your brain to stop eating when you're full, while ghrelin is a hormone that stimulates appetite. Insulin is another hormone that affects weight loss, as it helps regulate blood sugar levels and can impact feelings of hunger and satiety. Other factors that can influence weight loss include sleep quality, stress levels, and even the types of bacteria living in your gut. By understanding these various factors and how they contribute to weight management, you can create a more personalized approach to your weight loss journey that takes into account your unique needs and challenges.

In the next chapters, we'll explore each of these topics in more detail, delving into actionable strategies for creating a calorie deficit, optimizing your metabolism, and building healthy habits that support long-term success. By taking a science-backed, holistic approach to weight loss, you'll be better equipped to achieve your goals and maintain your results over time.

Chapter 3

Strategies for Creating a Calorie Deficit

Creating a calorie deficit is a critical component of successful weight loss. But many people struggle to know where to start when it comes to managing their food intake. In this chapter, we'll explore practical strategies for creating a calorie deficit that work for your lifestyle and preferences.

1. Track your food intake: Keeping a food diary or using a mobile app to track your meals and snacks can be a helpful way to become more mindful of your food choices and portion sizes and identify areas where you might be consuming too many calories without realizing it.

2. Focus on nutrient-dense, whole foods: As we mentioned earlier, prioritizing nutrient-dense, whole foods can help you feel fuller and more satisfied with fewer calories. Focus on lean proteins, fruits and vegetables, whole grains, and healthy fats.

3. Choose the right portion sizes: Understanding appropriate portion sizes can be a key strategy for achieving a calorie deficit. Use visual cues like your hand or measuring cups to help you gauge appropriate serving sizes based on your individual needs.

4. Plan ahead: When it comes to weight loss, failing to plan is planning to fail. By planning out your meals and snacks in advance, you can avoid impulse eating and ensure that you're providing your body with the nutrients it needs to thrive.

5. Don't skip meals: Many people assume that skipping meals is an effective way to lose weight, but in reality, it can lead to binging and overeating later on. Aim to eat three meals per day, with healthy snacks as needed, to keep your metabolism running smoothly.

6. Limit liquid calories: Sugary drinks like soda, juice, and energy drinks can add hundreds of unnecessary calories to your diet each day. Stick with water, unsweetened tea and coffee, and nutrient-rich smoothies with minimal added sugar.

7. Practice mindful eating: Mindful eating involves paying close attention to the sensory experience of your food, including the taste, texture, and aroma. By savoring your food and tuning into your body's hunger and fullness cues, you can avoid overeating and make more conscious food choices.

By incorporating these and other practical strategies into your weight loss plan, you can create a sustainable calorie deficit that promotes long-term success. In the next chapter, we'll explore the role of exercise in weight loss and how to create an effective fitness plan that complements your nutrition goals.

Chapter 4

The Role of Exercise in Weight Loss

While creating a calorie deficit through nutrition is essential for weight loss, exercise can also play a key role in achieving your goals. In this chapter, we'll explore the science of exercise for weight loss and how to create an effective workout plan that meets your needs.

First, it's important to understand how exercise contributes to weight loss. When you engage in physical activity, your body burns calories to fuel the activity. Over time, consistent exercise can help you build lean muscle mass, which increases your metabolism and helps you burn more calories even when you're at rest. However, not all exercises are created equal when it comes to weight loss. High-intensity interval training (HIIT), for example, has been found to be particularly effective for burning calories and boosting metabolism. Resistance training, such as weight lifting or bodyweight exercises, can also be effective for building muscle mass and improving body composition. Another key factor to consider when creating an exercise plan for weight loss is how much time you have available. The American Heart Association recommends at least 150 minutes of moderate-intensity aerobic activity or 75 minutes of vigorous-intensity aerobic activity per week for overall health benefits. However, if weight loss is your primary goal, you may need to increase your exercise volume to see significant results.

Here are some additional strategies for creating an effective exercise plan for weight loss:

1. Incorporate variety: Mixing up your workouts can help prevent boredom, prevent plateaus, and target different muscle groups. Try a combination of cardio, strength training, and flexibility exercises to keep your routine fresh and challenging.

2. Set realistic goals: Be honest with yourself about your current fitness level and set realistic goals based on your abilities. Gradually increasing the intensity and duration of your workouts over time can help you avoid injury and burnout.

3. Find accountability: Working out with a partner or hiring a personal trainer can help you stay motivated and committed to your fitness goals.

4. Prioritize recovery: Getting enough rest, staying hydrated, and eating a balanced diet can all help you recover from workouts and stay energized for your next workout.

By incorporating these and other exercise strategies into your weight loss plan, you can optimize your calorie-burning potential and improve your overall health and wellness. In the next chapter, we'll explore how to build healthy habits that support long-term weight loss success.

Chapter 5

Building Healthy Habits for Long-Term Success

Effective weight loss is about more than just counting calories and hitting the gym. It also requires building healthy habits and making lifestyle changes that support your goals. In this chapter, we'll explore strategies for creating healthy habits that promote long-term weight loss success.

1. Focus on progress, not perfection: No one is perfect, and it's important to approach your weight loss journey with a growth mindset, embracing your setbacks and using them as an opportunity to learn and grow. Celebrate your progress along the way, even if it's slow and steady.

2. Create a supportive environment: Surrounding yourself with people who support your weight loss goals and creating an environment that fosters healthy habits can be critical to long-term success. This might mean finding a workout buddy, stocking up on healthy foods, or joining a support group.

3. Practice self-care: Prioritizing self-care activities like mindfulness, relaxation, and stress reduction can help you stay focused and motivated on your weight loss goals. Daily practices like meditation, yoga, or journaling can help you cultivate a positive mindset and manage stress more effectively.

4. Set realistic expectations: True weight loss success takes time. Setting goals that are unrealistic or too aggressive can set you up for disappointment and frustration. Instead, focus on steady progress and sustainable lifestyle changes that will support your long-term health and wellness.

5. Get enough sleep: Research has shown that getting adequate sleep is essential for weight loss and weight management. Prioritize getting at least seven hours of quality sleep per night to support your body's natural processes and reduce stress levels.

6. Avoid extremes: It can be tempting to try extreme diets or workout programs in pursuit of rapid weight loss, but these approaches are rarely sustainable in the long term. Instead, aim for a balanced, moderate approach that promotes overall health and well-being.

By incorporating these strategies into your weight loss plan, you can cultivate a lifestyle that supports your goals and creates lasting change. Remember, weight loss is a journey, not a destination, and it's never too late to start taking steps toward a healthier, happier you.

Chapter 6

Overcoming Common Obstacles to Weight Loss

As with any worthwhile endeavor, there will be obstacles

and challenges along the way to achieving your weight loss goals. Being aware of these obstacles and how to overcome them can help you stay on track and stay motivated. In this chapter, we'll explore some common obstacles to weight loss and strategies for overcoming them.

1. Emotional eating: Many people turn to food for comfort, stress relief, or as a coping mechanism. Learning techniques for managing stress and negative emotions and finding alternatives to emotional eating can be an effective way to curb this behavior.

2. Plateaus: It's not uncommon to experience a plateau in weight loss progress, where your weight loss slows or stops altogether. Being patient and persistent, and adjusting your diet and exercise routine if necessary, can help you overcome this obstacle.

3. Self-sabotage: Negative self-talk or self-sabotaging behaviors can hold us back from reaching our goals. Practicing self-compassion, reframing negative thoughts, and setting small, achievable goals can help you overcome these tendencies.

4. Lack of motivation: Losing weight can be a challenging journey, and it's natural to experience fluctuations in motivation. Reconnecting with your "why," setting new goals, or seeking support from friends or family members can help reignite your motivation.

5. Social pressures: Social situations can be challenging for those trying to lose weight, especially if friends or family members are not supportive or encouraging. Learning to set boundaries, communicate your needs, and finding supportive communities online or in person can help you navigate these situations.

6. Physical barriers: Physical challenges like injuries or chronic health conditions can make exercise and healthy eating more difficult. Consulting with a healthcare provider or a registered dietitian, and finding modified exercises or activities that work for your body, can help you overcome these obstacles.

By being aware of these obstacles and implementing strategies to overcome them, you can stay committed to your weight loss goals and achieve long-term success. Remember, weight loss is an ongoing journey, and it's never too late to start improving your health and well-being.

Conclusion

Celebrating Your Weight Loss Success

Losing weight is a journey that requires patience, perseverance, and dedication. By incorporating healthy eating habits, exercise routines, and healthy lifestyle changes into your daily routine, you can achieve your weight loss goals and create lasting change. Remember, weight loss success is not just about the number on the scale – it's about improving your overall health and well-being. By focusing on progress, not perfection, cultivating self-care practices, and overcoming common obstacles, you can create a happier, healthier, and more fulfilling life.

So take a moment to celebrate your weight loss success, no matter how big or small. And remember, the journey doesn't end with weight loss – it's an ongoing process of self-improvement and self-discovery. By continuing to make healthy choices and prioritize your well-being, you can achieve long-term success and create a life that truly reflects your best self.

We hope this book has given you the tools, knowledge, and inspiration you need to start your weight loss journey and achieve the healthy lifestyle you deserve. Congratulations on taking this important step toward becoming your best self!